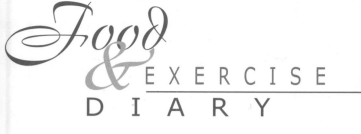

Food & EXERCISE DIARY

Introduction

The food diary is the most powerful proven aid for dieters. Persons who keep a food and exercise diary not only lose more weight they also keep it off. Here are some of the reasons:

▶ **Recording your eating and exercise habits** jolts you into realizing just what you do eat and drink each day; and also whether you exercise sufficiently.

▶ **Helps you identify problem foods** and drinks with excessive calories and fat.

▶ **Helps identify moods**, situations and events that lead to excessive eating of unwanted calories. You can then plan to overcome or avoid them.

▶ **Prevents 'calorie amnesia'**, the forgetful~~ss that~~ leads to rebound weight gain after s weight loss. Recording puts you back o track.

▶ **Helps you develop greater self-disciplin** think twice about over-indulging if y record it - especially if someone checks regularly. It certainly keeps you hones

▶ **Motivates you** to carefully plan your to exercise each day.

▶ **Serves as a check system** for your docto or counselor to assess your progress recommendations.

HOW TO USE THIS DIARY

1. **(a) Record your starting weight and measurements** on the 'Progress Chart' (Page 96). Ideally, also have your blood pressure, blood cholesterol and blood glucose checked.

(b) Set a goal or target weight loss that you wish to attain or maintain over the next 10 weeks. Be realistic. An average weight loss of 1-2 lbs per week is ideal. The heavier your starting weight, the greater the initial weight loss is likely to be.

(c) Decide on a calorie level that will allow a gradual weight loss. Suggested calorie ranges for weight loss are:

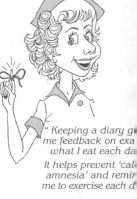

Women:	1000-1500 Calories
Men:	1200-1800 Calories
Children:	1000-1500 Calories
Teenagers:	1200-1800 Calories

Note: People who should not diet strictly unless medically supervised include: infants, pregnant or breastfeeding women, and persons with diabetes (on insulin).

" Keeping a diary g[ives]
me feedback on exa[ctly]
what I eat each da[y]

It helps prevent 'cal[orie]
amnesia' and remi[nds]
me to exercise each d[ay]

2. **Record all foods and drinks consumed. Calculate calories and fat.** Weigh food portions whenever possible in order to calculate calories and fat more accurately. With experience you will soon be able to estimate the calories and fat of foods most commonly eaten, without having to weigh them each time. Be sure to include all drinks and snacks. Round to the nearest 10 calories and one gram of fat.
NOTE: Record carbohydrate or protein if directed by your counselor.

3. **Record your exercise each day.** Record the number of minutes of physical activity over and above your regular daily routine. Aim for an extra 30-40 minutes of brisk walking or activity each day. Ideally, aim to burn an extra 250 - 500 exercise calories. Calculate exercise calories using the following simplified chart. Round to the nearest 10 calories.

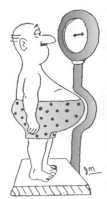

Abdominal obesity is a health-hazard, more so if not physically fit

LIGHT EXERCISE 4 Calories/Minute	MODERATE 7 Calories/Minute	HEAVY EXERCISE 10 Calories/Minute
Walking, Slow	Walking, Brisk	Walking(power), Jogging
Gardening, light	Aerobics, light	Aerobics, advanced
Cycling, light	Cycling, moderate	Cycling, strenuous
Calisthenics	Swimming, Aquarobics	Swimming, strenuous
Golf, social	Weight-training, light	Weight-training, heavy
Tennis, doubles	Tennis, singles	Wrestling/ Judo, advanced
Housework, light	Racquetball, beginners	Racketball, advanced
Ten Pin Bowls	Football	Football, training
Table Tennis, social	Basketball, Baseball	Basketball (Pro)
Horse-riding	Walking Downstairs	Climbing Stairs, Skipping
Ice Skating	Snow Skiing (downhill)	Snow Skiing (Cross-country)
Skate Boarding	Line/Square Dancing	Tae Bo, Kick Boxing
Yoga, Tai Chi	Dancing, Jazzercize	Dancing, strenuous

Note: Only those sports or activities that are sustained over a period of time (e.g. running) qualify
for heavy exercise. Stop-start sports such as tennis are considered 'moderate' on average.

4. At the end of each day:

(a) **Total each column** for 'Food Calories' and
'Exercise Calories.'

(b) **Deduct 'Exercise Calories' from 'Food Calories.'**
This determines your net calorie intake for
the day.

(c) **Total the 'Fat' column.** as well as carbohydrate
or protein if required.

5. At the end of each week:

(a) **Transfer the daily results** to the 'Weekly
Summary' page.

(b) **Calculate the daily average** of net calories and
fat. Simply add up the 7 days and divide by 7.

(c) **Transfer the average of the 'Weekly Summary'**
to the 'Progress Chart' on the last page of
the diary.

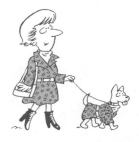

Exercising 3-4 times weekly
may be fine for aerobic
fitness but daily
exercise is a must for
effective weight control.

Sample Recording

		CALORIES		FAT	CARBS or
		Food	Exercise	Grams	Protein
☺ BREAKFAST/Exercise	Brisk Walk, 20mins		140		
	1 cup Wheatbran Flakes	110		1	25
	1 Tbsp Wheatgerm	30		1	4
	1 Tbsp Sunflower Seeds	45		4	2
	½ large Banana, sliced	60		0	12
	¾ cup Milk (1% Fat)	80		2	9
Snack/Exercise					
☺ LUNCH	2 thin slices Wholewheat Bread	140		2	26
	3 tsp Light Margarine	50		6	0
	½ small Avocado	90		9	3
	2 Tbsp Ricotta Cheese (part-skim)	40		3	1
	1 medium Tomato	30		0	6
	Lettuce; Bean Sprouts	10		0	2
Snack/Exercise	1 medium Apple	90		0	23
	Exercise Bike, 10 min		70		
☺ DINNER	Vegetable Soup (fat-free)	40		0	9
	Broiled Fish, 5 oz	160		2	0
	1 tsp light Margarine	20		2	0
	½ cup Broccoli, 3 oz	25		0	5
	½ cup Carrots	35		0	8
	1 small Potato, 3 oz	65		0	15
Snack/Exercise	1 medium Orange	70		0	17
	Diet Gelatine + Fruit Salad	50		0	11
	2 cups Popcorn (plain), ½ oz	50		0	10
	Diet Drink	0		0	0
Mon CALORIE TOTALS		1290	210		
NET CALORIES (Food Minus Exercise)		1080			

WATER/FLUIDS (CUPS) 🥛🥛🥛🥛🥛🥛🥛🥛
Includes juice/Milk/Soup

Total Fat (Grams) 32g

Total Carbohydrate 188g

Steps (Pedometer): 8,500

Comments & Resolutions:

PAGE 4   *A reasonable day ~ felt in control*   ©

TEN DIETING HINTS

1. Avoid fad diets. They don't re-educate your eating habits. Eat 3 moderate meals daily that are nutritionally balanced. Drink adequate fluids.

2. Carefully plan each meal rather than just grabbing haphazardly whatever comes into your line of vision. Use a shopping list at supermarkets.

3. Don't skip meals. You are more likely to snack on high calorie, high-fat foods.

4. Use minimal amounts of fat and oil. Trim fat from meat, and skin from poultry. Use low-fat dairy products and low-fat salad dressings. Use fat-free cooking methods. Avoid fried foods, high-fat snacks and high-fat fast foods, cookies, cakes and icecream. Limit nuts. (Extra notes ~ see Page 8-9)

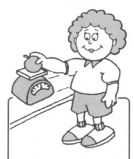

Weigh your food until you can accurately estimate food portion sizes. Better control of calories will result

5. Avoid sugar and foods high in sugar such as sodas, fruit drinks, jams, chocolate, cookies, cakes, icecream and ice confections. Use sugar substitutes and sugar-free diet products.

6. Eat at least 5 serves of fruits and vegetables each day. Also eat wholegrain cereal products. They are nutritious and help to prevent constipation.

7. There is no food that cannot occasionally be eaten, for example chocolate, cake, dessert, wine. It is the quantity that is critical. Total deprivation can lead to binge eating.

8. Avoid alcohol when dieting. Avoid regular sodas; use sugar-free diet drinks. Limit fruit juice. Be sure to drink adequate water.

9. When dining out, avoid fried and sauce-laden dishes as well as pastries, regular salad dressings and desserts. Eat moderately. Quench your thirst on water, mineral water or low calorie diet drinks.

10. Take a multi-vitamin and mineral supplement when dieting, particularly if tired and irritable.

For online support, food product updates and healthy recipes, see www.calorieking.com

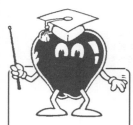

Eating a high fiber breakfast gives you a good start to the day ...and helps prevent high calorie snacking.

Desirable lower calorie snacks include apples, oranges, carrot sticks and plain popcorn.

CARBOHYDRATES

- **Carbohydrate foods** in their more natural forms are an important part of a healthy diet. They provide energy, fiber, vitamins, minerals, protein and water. They are found mainly in cereal grains, fruit, vegetables and milk. Meats, diary and eggs contain no fiber.

  A healthy diet of at least 2000 calories is based around carbohydrate foods and should provide over 50% of total calories. Lower calorie diets for weight loss should still have around 40% of total calories from carbohydrates.

- **Carbohydrates include** sugars, starches and fiber. Sugars and starch provide energy to body cells. Even though fiber is not digested, it benefits the body.

Carbohydrate Intake Guide

Daily Total Calories		Daily Total Carbohyd.	Percent Carbohyd. Cals
▼		▼	▼
1200 Cals	~	120g	40%
1500 Cals	~	170g	45%
2000 Cals	~	250g	50%
2500 Cals	~	345g	55%
3000 Cals	~	450g	60%

LOW CARBOHYDRATE FAD DIETS

Some fad diets encourage carbohydrate intake to be drastically cut as low as 20 grams per day; and claim that you can eat as much meat, protein, fat and calories as you wish. Such diets can be decidedly unhealthy.

Health experts advise a minimum carbohydrate intake of 100 grams per day. Well-balanced diets for weight loss are already reduced in carbohydrate without going to the extreme. Weight from fat stores will only be lost if calorie intake is less than the body requires.

Large initial weight losses on fad diets are mainly due to body fluid losses.

DIABETES & CARBOHYDRATES

- **For people with diabetes**, regular meals with even distribution of carbohydrate over the day are important for good control of blood sugar levels.

- **Smaller amounts of food** eaten more frequently result in steadier, more even blood glucose levels. (Be sure to control your weight.)

- For persons with diabetes who are on insulin, distribution of carbohydrate intake should be over three main meals as well as between-meal snacks (if directed by your counselor).

- **Your doctor or dietitian** will select the level of calories and carbohydrate most appropriate to your weight, medication and activity. (Regular blood glucose checks will provide feedback on the level of control.)

- **Total daily carbohydrate** should provide around 50% of total calories.

  A **rough rule of thumb is:** 13 grams of carbohydrate per 100 calories.

  At calorie levels above 2000, carbohydrates approach 50-60% of total calories.

  At lower calorie levels used for weight loss (1200-1500 calories), carbohydrates account for as little as 40% of total calories. This is because protein has nutritional priority.

  These carbohydrate quantities apply equally to persons with or without diabetes.

FIBER IS HEALTHY!

Eating high-fiber foods (whole-grain bread and cereals, beans, nuts, seeds, fruits, veggies) benefits blood glucose control and general health.

RECOMMENDED FAT INTAKE

FAT IN THE DIET

- Fats in the diet are essential for good health. However, too much fat can contribute to obesity, and a higher risk of heart disease, high blood pressure, diabetes, gallstones and certain cancers.

- Dietary fats/oils have over double the calories of carbohydrates and protein:

CALORIE VALUES PER GRAM

Carbohydrate:	~	4 Calories
Protein:	~	4 Calories
Fat/Oil:	~	9 Calories
Alcohol:	~	7 Calories

- **Dietary fat** is more readily converted to and stored as body fat compared to carbohydrates and protein.

- **Excess carbohydrates** over body needs may also be converted and stored as body fat - especially in women in their fertile years when extra fat pads are more readily laid down in the thighs and buttocks.

- **Excess alcohol** lessens the body's ability to burn fat. Fat storage is promoted, particularly in the belly - a danger zone.

RECOMMENDED FAT INTAKE

Americans consume too much fat with many having over 40% of total calories from fat - either as fat or oil, or as fat in foods and drinks A range of 20-30% is considered to be much healthier.

Healthy Ranges for Fat Intake:

Children	~	30-60g
Teenagers (Active)	~	40-80g
Women	~	30-60g
Men: Active	~	40-80g
Heavy Activity/Athlete	~	80-120g

The chart below shows the recommended maximum fat intake for different energy levels.

INFANTS FAT INTAKE

Infants and toddlers under 3 years should not be restricted in their fat intake because much larger volumes of food would be required to guarantee adequate calories and growth. Whole milk should be used rather than low-fat milk (1%) or nonfat milk.

Similarly, a high fiber diet is also not suitable for infants.

MAXIMUM DESIRABLE FAT INTAKE

CALORIES ▼	FAT ▼	% Cals From FAT ▼
1200 cals	30g fat	23%
1500 cals	40g fat	24%
1800 cals	50g fat	25%
2000 cals	60g fat	27%
2200 cals	70g fat	28%
2500 cals	80g fat	29%
2800 cals	90g fat	29%
3000 cals	100g fat	30%
3500 cals	117g fat	30%
4000 cals	135g fat	30%

HINTS TO REDUCE FAT

MEATS & POULTRY

- **Choose lean cuts** of meat with little marbling. Choose the white meat of chicken and turkey, and extra lean ground beef.
- **Trim all visible fat** from meat and remove the skin from poultry.
- **Eat modest portions** (3-4 oz cooked weight) of meat, poultry or fish. **Add extra** beans, lentils, tofu, tempeh, vegetables, potatoes, rice, bread.
- **Avoid high-fat meat products** such as sausages, bacon, salami and other cold cuts. Choose lower-fat varieties. Check the nutritional panel on the label.
- **Broil or bake.** Avoid frying. Allow casseroles to cool and skim off any surface fat.

FISH & SEAFOODS

- **Choose fresh or frozen fillets,** canned fish (in water pack).
- **Avoid fried fish,** frozen fish in batter, canned fish in oil.

FATS, OILS, CREAM

- **Use minimal amounts** of all types of fat and oil. All are high in calories.
  Note: While healthier, vegetable oils and spreads have the same calories as solid shortenings and animal fats.
- **Cream:** Avoid cream, sour cream and powdered coffee creamers.
- **Use yogurt in place of cream** in recipes.
- Use as little fat as possible to cook vegetables and grain products.
- **Use minimal amounts of oil** when stir-frying. Use oil sprays such as *Pam*.

SALAD DRESSINGS & SAUCES

- **Limit mayonnaise and oil dressings.** Choose low-oil or no-oil dressings (e.g. *Kraft Free, Hidden Valley Ranch, Pritikin*).
- **Choose low-fat sauces** to accompany pasta, rice and potatoes.

MILK & DAIRY; SOY DRINKS

- **Choose** low-fat or skim milks; and yogurts. Avoid full-cream milk, cream, *Half & Half* coffee creamers.
- **Soy Drinks:** Choose low-fat brands.
- **Cheese:** Choose low-fat and fat-reduced such as cottage and low-fat ricotta. Cheese substitutes can still be high in fat.
- **Icecream:** Choose low-fat ice milks, frozen yogurt, sorbet, sherbet and ices. Limit regular icecream to a small serving. Avoid rich high-fat icecreams.

FROZEN ENTREES & MEALS

- **Choose low-fat varieties** such as *Lean Cuisine, Healthy Choice and Weight Watchers.* Supplement them with extra vegetables or salads and fruit.

FRYING ADDS FAT!

The greater the surface area of potato exposed to fat or oil, the higher the fat content.

Whole Potato (3 oz)
Nil Fat, 65 Cals

Roast Potato (3 oz)
8g fat, 125 Cals

French Fries
Large Cut (3 oz)
12g fat, 220 Cals

French Fries
Small Cut (3 oz)
15g fat, 275 Cals

Potato Chips (3 oz)
30g fat, 450 Cals

HINTS TO REDUCE FAT

BREADS, BAGELS, CRACKERS

- **All breads are suitable** as well as pita, bagels, English muffins and rice cakes. Avoid croissants, sweet rolls, danish pastry fat-soaked toast and garlic toast.
- **Choose low-fat crackers** such as graham, saltines, matzo, bread sticks, crispbreads. Avoid cheese or butter crackers.

CEREALS, PASTA, RICE

- **Most** hot and cold cereals are low in fat. Choose ones with less than 3g fat per serve.
- **Choose** plain pasta or rice. **Avoid** dishes made with cream, butter or cheese sauces.

FRUITS & VEGETABLES

- **Choose all types.** Use minimal fat or oil in cooking. Mashed avocado is a suitable replacement on bread in place of fat.
- **Choose** dried beans, lentils, chick peas, baked beans.
- **Avoid** french-fried potatoes, hash browns, and regular potato salad. **Avoid** vegetables made in butter, cream or sauce. Use minimal oil when stir frying.
- **Avoid** deli-style salads made with high-fat dressings.

SNACKS, COOKIES & CANDY

- **Avoid** high-fat snacks such as potato chips, corn/tortilla chips, *Chee-Tos, Cheez Balls,* buttered popcorn, chocolate and carbo bars.
- **Avoid** donuts. cakes, cookies, pastries
- **Choose** plain popcorn, low-fat cookies and muffins, hard candy, jelly beans, fruit rolls and frozen fruit popsicles. Limit quantities.
- **Choose** fresh and dried fruits, vegetables. Limit nuts and seeds if overweight.
- **Choose** low-fat vegetable or noodle soups. Most *Cup-A-Soup* varieties are suitable.
- **Avoid** ramen noodle cup meals.

DESSERTS/SWEETS

- **Avoid high-fat desserts,** such as fruit pies, pastries, cheesecake, cheeseboard.
- **Choose** fresh fruits, fresh fruit salad, low-fat custard, yogurt, frozen yogurt, sorbet. Use yogurt in place of cream or icecream.

FAST-FOODS & TAKE OUT

- **Deli's:** Choose sandwiches/bread rolls, pitas with low-fat fillings and plain salad. Limit meat/cheese to small portions. Avoid high-fat deli salads. Choose plain salads and add your own low-fat dressing. Eat more fruit.
- **Chicken & Fish:** Avoid deep-fried chicken or fish, BBQ chicken with fat or skin, chicken nuggets. Choose broiled or baked chicken breast and discard the skin.
- **Hamburgers:** Choose medium size, lower fat burgers. Avoid bacon. Have a side salad (with low-calorie dressing).
- **Pizzas:** Avoid sausage/pepperoni. Choose vegetarian topping and modest quantity of cheese. Eat a moderate serving. Eat extra salad and fruit.
- **French Fries and Potatoes:** Avoid french fries and fried onion rings. Choose whole roast or baked potatoes (butter or sour cream on the side) or, replace fries with salad, coleslaw, bean salad, corn peas.
- **Desserts & Drinks:** Avoid apple pie, danish, choc chip cookies and soda. Choose low-fat muffins *(eg. McDonald's)* frozen yogurt, fruit salad and orange juice. Limit to small serving.
- **Restaurant Chains:** Choose 'lite' menu dishes. They can cut up to 75% of the fat off regular dishes. Avoid deep-fried or battered and fried dishes. Check the above notes.

- Persons who exercise regularly lose more weight and keep it off longer than non-exercisers.

- Exercise also improves general health and well-being. Confidence and self-esteem are enhanced by a sense of control and accomplishment.

- Dieting alone results in a loss of both body fat and muscle, whereas exercise and strength training results in loss of mainly body fat. Building or maintaining muscles aids body reshaping and increases the body's metabolic rate (allowing you to eat more food).

Note: When fat is lost and muscle gained, there may be little change in weight. Yet fatness has been reduced as evidenced by a smaller size of clothing fitting the reproportioned body. Weight from exercised muscles is okay. It is surplus fat that is potentially harmful.

- **Exercise increases the metabolic rate** of the body even for hours after exercise. A good way to 'wake up' a sluggish metabolism.

  Exercise compensates for any decrease in metabolic rate with increasing age and also in some heavy smokers who stop smoking.

- **Avoid injury** by beginning with walking, low impact aerobics, or weight-supported exercise (e.g. swimming, cycling). Avoid competitive sports.

- **How Much?** Start with 10 - 20 minutes a day and progress to 30-45 minutes a day.

  Also walk up stairs instead of using lifts. Take a brisk walk at lunch. Use an exercise bike, treadmill or stepper while watching TV.

- **How Often?** While aerobic fitness requires only 3 - 4 sessions weekly, **weight control is a daily event which requires daily exercise.**

TV CAN BE FATTENING!

Many adults and children watch over 20 hours of television per week (in addition to computer games and internet surfing); and indulge in high-fat snacks at the same time - potent contributors to obesity.
Are you a TV couch potato? Limit your TV and computer hours and plan healthy physical activities.

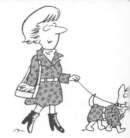

Brisk walking each day is a s and effective way to keep tri and fit. Try it - you'll like it!

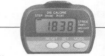

Use a pedometer to count your steps each day.
It motivates you to keep moving
Aim for 10,000 steps daily.
Extra info: www.calorieking.com

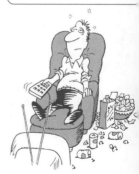

Daily exercise and sensible eating can prevent middle-age spread.

EATING BEHAVIOR

- Eating is a behavior that is largely controlled by people with whom we live or socialize, places in which we carry out our lives, and our emotions. Become aware of those situations that commonly lead to extra food being eaten.

- We may also be unaware of 'bad' eating habits that can lead to excess calorie intake; e.g. eating quickly, large mouthsful, eating when tense or bored, finishing a large serving of food when not hungry.

Hints to help uncover and correct those 'bad' eating habits include:

- **Don't eat while engaged in other activities;** e.g. watching TV, reading. Eat only at the table, not at the fridge or while standing.

- **Don't eat quickly.** Chewing slowly allows time to register a feeling of fullness. Don't use fingers, only utensils. Cut food into smaller pieces. Don't load your fork until the previous mouthful is finished.

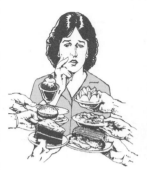

Practise saying 'NO' politely but assertively.

- **Don't purchase problem high calorie foods.** Shop from a set list to prevent impulse buying. Avoid shopping with children. Plan meals in advance. Stick to a set menu.

- **Plan a strategy to avoid uncontrolled eating** and drinking at social events, or when your emotions urge you to binge.

Rehearse repeatedly in your mind exactly what you will do in such situations. Remind yourself several times each day that you are in charge of your actions and that you can be strong-willed. Seek counseling or coaching on various strategies.

- **Promise yourself** that when you feel the urge to snack, you will engage in some activity that will distract you away from food (e.g. go for a walk, brush your teeth, phone a friend.)

If you eat out of boredom, find some new hobby or interest that gets you out of the house. Even enroll in an adult education class.

Note:
- Persons with deep-seated emotional problems and eating disorders require counseling. See a doctor's referral to a specialist.

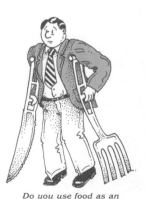

Do you use food as an emotional crutch?

If so, professional counseling may be helpful.

Monday

	CALORIES		FAT	CARBS or
	FOOD	EXERCISE	GRAMS	PROTEIN
🙂 BREAKFAST/Exercise				
Snack/Exercise				
🙂 LUNCH				
Snack/Exercise				
🙂 DINNER				
Snack/Exercise				
Mon CALORIE TOTALS				
NET CALORIES (Food Minus Exercise)				

WATER/FLUIDS (CUPS) ⛌ ⛌ ⛌ ⛌ ⛌ ⛌ ⛌ ⛌
Includes juice/Milk/Soup

Total Fat (Grams)
Total Carbohydrate

Steps (Pedometer):_ _ _ _ _ _ _ _ _ _ _

Comments & Resolutions:

©

Tuesday

	CALORIES		FAT	CARBS or PROTEIN
	FOOD	EXERCISE	GRAMS	
🙂 BREAKFAST/Exercise				
Snack/Exercise				
🙂 LUNCH				
Snack/Exercise				
🙂 DINNER				
Snack/Exercise				
CALORIE TOTALS				
Tue NET CALORIES (Food Minus Exercise)				

WATER/FLUIDS (CUPS) ⬜⬜⬜⬜⬜⬜⬜⬜
Includes juice/Milk/Soup

Total Fat (Grams)
Total Carbohydrate

Steps (Pedometer):_ _ _ _ _ _ _ _ _ _

Comments & Resolutions:

©

Wednesday

	CALORIES		FAT	CARBS or PROTEIN
	FOOD	EXERCISE	GRAMS	
😊 **BREAKFAST**/Exercise				
Snack/Exercise				
😊 **LUNCH**				
Snack/Exercise				
😊 **DINNER**				
Snack/Exercise				
Wed **CALORIE TOTALS**				
NET CALORIES (Food Minus Exercise)				

WATER/FLUIDS (CUPS) 🥛🥛🥛🥛🥛🥛🥛🥛
Includes juice/Milk/Soup

Total Fat (Grams)

Total Carbohydrate

Steps (Pedometer):_ _ _ _ _ _ _ _ _ _ _ _

Comments & Resolutions:

©

Thursday

	CALORIES		FAT	CARBS
	FOOD	EXERCISE	GRAMS	or PROTEIN
☺ **BREAKFAST**/Exercise				
Snack/Exercise				
☺ **LUNCH**				
Snack/Exercise				
☺ **DINNER**				
Snack/Exercise				
Thu **CALORIE TOTALS**				
NET CALORIES (Food Minus Exercise)				

WATER/FLUIDS (CUPS) ▽ ▽ ▽ ▽ ▽ ▽ ▽ ▽
Includes juice/Milk/Soup

Total Fat (Grams)	
Total Carbohydrate	

Steps (Pedometer): _ _ _ _ _ _ _ _ _ _

Comments & Resolutions:

©

	CALORIES		FAT	CARBS or PROTEIN
	FOOD	EXERCISE	GRAMS	

Friday

☺ **BREAKFAST/Exercise**

Snack/Exercise

☺ **LUNCH**

Snack/Exercise

☺ **DINNER**

Snack/Exercise

Fri CALORIE TOTALS				
NET CALORIES (Food Minus Exercise)				

WATER/FLUIDS (CUPS) ▽▽▽▽▽▽▽▽
Includes juice/Milk/Soup

Total Fat (Grams)

Total Carbohydrate

Steps (Pedometer): _ _ _ _ _ _ _ _ _ _ _

Comments & Resolutions:

©

Saturday

	CALORIES		FAT	CARBS or PROTEIN
	FOOD	EXERCISE	GRAMS	
☺ BREAKFAST/Exercise				
Snack/Exercise				
☺ LUNCH				
Snack/Exercise				
☺ DINNER				
Snack/Exercise				
Sat CALORIE TOTALS				
NET CALORIES (Food Minus Exercise)				

WATER/FLUIDS (CUPS) ▽ ▽ ▽ ▽ ▽ ▽ ▽ ▽
Includes juice/Milk/Soup

Total Fat (Grams)	
Total Carbohydrate	

Steps (Pedometer):_ _ _ _ _ _ _ _ _ _ _ _

Comments & Resolutions:

©

Sunday

	CALORIES		FAT	CARBS or
	FOOD	EXERCISE	GRAMS	PROTEIN
☺ BREAKFAST/Exercise				
Snack/Exercise				
☺ LUNCH				
Snack/Exercise				
☺ DINNER				
Snack/Exercise				
CALORIE TOTALS				
Sun **NET CALORIES** (Food Minus Exercise)				

WATER/FLUIDS (CUPS) ▽ ▽ ▽ ▽ ▽ ▽ ▽ ▽
Includes juice/Milk/Soup

Total Fat (Grams)

Total Carbohydrate

Steps (Pedometer):_ _ _ _ _ _ _ _ _ _ _ _

Comments & Resolutions:

©

WEEKLY SUMMARY

week **1**

Day	Net Calories	Fat Grams	Carbohydrates
Monday			
Tuesday			
Wednesday			
Thursday			
Friday			
Saturday			
Sunday			
WEEK'S TOTALS			
DAILY AVERAGES Divide totals by 7			

WEIGHT CHANGE

One week ago: _____

Today: _____

Weight Change: _____

WAIST CHANGE

One week ago: _____

Today: _____

Waist Change: _____

⊘ Transfer daily averages for calories and fat to last page.
⊘ Record body measurements on last page (chest, waist, hips, thighs).

COMMENTS :

_____

_____

GOALS / RESOLUTIONS FOR NEXT WEEK:

_____

_____

_____

Monday

| | CALORIES | | FAT | CARBS or |
	Food	Exercise	Grams	Protein
🙂 **BREAKFAST/Exercise**				
Snack/Exercise				
🙂 **LUNCH**				
Snack/Exercise				
🙂 **DINNER**				
Snack/Exercise				

	CALORIE TOTALS			
Mon NET CALORIES (Food Minus Exercise)				

WATER/FLUIDS (CUPS) ▽ ▽ ▽ ▽ ▽ ▽ ▽ ▽
Includes juice/Milk/Soup

| **Total Fat (Grams)** | |
| **Total Carbohydrate** | |

Steps (Pedometer): _ _ _ _ _ _ _ _ _ _ _ _

Comments & Resolutions:

©

Tuesday

| | CALORIES | | FAT | CARBS or |
	FOOD	EXERCISE	GRAMS	PROTEIN
☺ BREAKFAST/Exercise				
Snack/Exercise				
☺ LUNCH				
Snack/Exercise				
☺ DINNER				
Snack/Exercise				
Tue CALORIE TOTALS				
NET CALORIES (Food Minus Exercise)				

WATER/FLUIDS (CUPS) ▢ ▢ ▢ ▢ ▢ ▢ ▢ ▢
Includes juice/Milk/Soup

Total Fat (Grams)
Total Carbohydrate

Steps (Pedometer): _ _ _ _ _ _ _ _ _ _

Comments & Resolutions:

©

Wednesday

| | CALORIES | | FAT | CARBS or |
	Food	Exercise	Grams	Protein
😊 **BREAKFAST**/Exercise				
Snack/Exercise				
😊 **LUNCH**				
Snack/Exercise				
😊 **DINNER**				
Snack/Exercise				
CALORIE TOTALS				
NET CALORIES (Food Minus Exercise)				

Wed

WATER/FLUIDS (CUPS) ⛶ ⛶ ⛶ ⛶ ⛶ ⛶ ⛶ ⛶
Includes juice/Milk/Soup

Total Fat (Grams)
Total Carbohydrate

Steps (Pedometer): _ _ _ _ _ _ _ _ _ _ _ _

Comments & Resolutions:

©

Thursday

	CALORIES		FAT	CARBS or PROTEIN
	FOOD	EXERCISE	GRAMS	
☺ BREAKFAST/Exercise				
Snack/Exercise				
☺ LUNCH				
Snack/Exercise				
☺ DINNER				
Snack/Exercise				
CALORIE TOTALS				
NET CALORIES (Food Minus Exercise)				

Thu

WATER/FLUIDS (CUPS) Includes juice/Milk/Soup ▽▽▽▽▽▽▽▽

Total Fat (Grams)

Total Carbohydrate

Steps (Pedometer): _ _ _ _ _ _ _ _ _ _ _

Comments & Resolutions:

©

Friday

	CALORIES		FAT	CARBS or PROTEIN
	FOOD	EXERCISE	GRAMS	
🙂 **BREAKFAST/Exercise**				
Snack/Exercise				
🙂 **LUNCH**				
Snack/Exercise				
🙂 **DINNER**				
Snack/Exercise				
Fri CALORIE TOTALS				
NET CALORIES (Food Minus Exercise)				

WATER/FLUIDS (CUPS) ⬜⬜⬜⬜⬜⬜⬜
Includes juice/Milk/Soup

Total Fat (Grams)

Total Carbohydrate

Steps (Pedometer):_ _ _ _ _ _ _ _ _ _ _

Comments & Resolutions:

©

Saturday

| | CALORIES | | FAT | CARBS |
	FOOD	EXERCISE	GRAMS	or PROTEIN
☺ BREAKFAST/Exercise				
Snack/Exercise				
☺ LUNCH				
Snack/Exercise				
☺ DINNER				
Snack/Exercise				
Sat CALORIE TOTALS				
NET CALORIES (Food Minus Exercise)				

WATER/FLUIDS (CUPS) ▽ ▽ ▽ ▽ ▽ ▽ ▽ ▽
Includes juice/Milk/Soup

Total Fat (Grams)

Total Carbohydrate

Steps (Pedometer): _ _ _ _ _ _ _ _ _ _

Comments & Resolutions:

©

Sunday

| | CALORIES | | FAT | CARBS or |
	FOOD	EXERCISE	GRAMS	PROTEIN
🙂 **BREAKFAST/Exercise**				
Snack/Exercise				
🙂 **LUNCH**				
Snack/Exercise				
🙂 **DINNER**				
Snack/Exercise				
CALORIE TOTALS				
NET CALORIES (Food Minus Exercise)				

WATER/FLUIDS (CUPS) ▽▽▽▽▽▽▽▽
Includes juice/Milk/Soup

Total Fat (Grams)

Total Carbohydrate

Steps (Pedometer):_ _ _ _ _ _ _ _ _ _ _

Comments & Resolutions:

PAGE 26   ©

WEEKLY SUMMARY

week 2

Day	Net Calories	Fat Grams	Carbohydrates
Monday			
Tuesday			
Wednesday			
Thursday			
Friday			
Saturday			
Sunday			
WEEK'S TOTALS			
DAILY AVERAGES Divide totals by 7			

WEIGHT CHANGE

One week ago: _____

Today: _____

Weight Change: _____

WAIST CHANGE

One week ago: _____

Today: _____

Waist Change: _____

⊘ Transfer daily averages for calories and fat to last page.
⊘ Record body measurements on last page (chest, waist, hips, thighs).

COMMENTS :
_____
_____
_____

GOALS / RESOLUTIONS FOR NEXT WEEK:
_____
_____
_____

©

Monday

| | CALORIES | | FAT | CARBS or |
	Food	Exercise	Grams	Protein
☺ **BREAKFAST**/Exercise				
Snack/Exercise				
☺ **LUNCH**				
Snack/Exercise				
☺ **DINNER**				
Snack/Exercise				
CALORIE TOTALS				
NET CALORIES (Food Minus Exercise)				

Mon

WATER/FLUIDS (CUPS) ▽ ▽ ▽ ▽ ▽ ▽ ▽ ▽
Includes juice/Milk/Soup

| **Total Fat (Grams)** | |
| **Total Carbohydrate** | |

Steps (Pedometer): _ _ _ _ _ _ _ _ _ _ _ _

Comments & Resolutions:

PAGE 28

©

Tuesday

	CALORIES		FAT	CARBS or
	FOOD	EXERCISE	GRAMS	PROTEIN
☺ BREAKFAST/Exercise				
Snack/Exercise				
☺ LUNCH				
Snack/Exercise				
☺ DINNER				
Snack/Exercise				
CALORIE TOTALS				
NET CALORIES (Food Minus Exercise)				

WATER/FLUIDS (CUPS) ▯ ▯ ▯ ▯ ▯ ▯ ▯ ▯
Includes juice/Milk/Soup

Total Fat (Grams)

Total Carbohydrate

Steps (Pedometer):_ _ _ _ _ _ _ _ _ _ _ _

Comments & Resolutions:

©

Wednesday

	CALORIES		FAT	CARBS or
	Food	Exercise	Grams	Protein
😊 BREAKFAST/Exercise				
Snack/Exercise				
😊 LUNCH				
Snack/Exercise				
😊 DINNER				
Snack/Exercise				
CALORIE TOTALS				
NET CALORIES (Food Minus Exercise)				

WATER/FLUIDS (CUPS) ⬆ ⬆ ⬆ ⬆ ⬆ ⬆ ⬆
Includes juice/Milk/Soup

Total Fat (Grams)	
Total Carbohydrate	

Steps (Pedometer): _ _ _ _ _ _ _ _ _ _ _ _

Comments & Resolutions:

©

Thursday

| | CALORIES | | FAT | CARBS |
	FOOD	EXERCISE	GRAMS	or PROTEIN
☺ **BREAKFAST**/Exercise				
Snack/Exercise				
☺ **LUNCH**				
Snack/Exercise				
☺ **DINNER**				
Snack/Exercise				
Thu CALORIE TOTALS				
NET CALORIES (Food Minus Exercise)				

WATER/FLUIDS (CUPS) ▽ ▽ ▽ ▽ ▽ ▽ ▽ ▽
Includes juice/Milk/Soup

| **Total Fat (Grams)** |
| **Total Carbohydrate** |

Steps (Pedometer):_ _ _ _ _ _ _ _ _ _ _

Comments & Resolutions:

©

Friday

	CALORIES		FAT	CARBS or
	FOOD	EXERCISE	GRAMS	PROTEIN
☺ BREAKFAST/Exercise				
Snack/Exercise				
☺ LUNCH				
Snack/Exercise				
☺ DINNER				
Snack/Exercise				
Fri CALORIE TOTALS				
NET CALORIES (Food Minus Exercise)				

WATER/FLUIDS (CUPS) ▽ ▽ ▽ ▽ ▽ ▽ ▽
Includes juice/Milk/Soup

Total Fat (Grams)
Total Carbohydrate

Steps (Pedometer):_ _ _ _ _ _ _ _ _ _ _ _

Comments & Resolutions:

©

Saturday

| | CALORIES | | FAT | CARBS |
	FOOD	EXERCISE	GRAMS	or PROTEIN
🙂 **BREAKFAST**/Exercise				
Snack/Exercise				
🙂 **LUNCH**				
Snack/Exercise				
🙂 **DINNER**				
Snack/Exercise				
Sat **CALORIE TOTALS**				
NET CALORIES (Food Minus Exercise)				

WATER/FLUIDS (CUPS) ⛾ ⛾ ⛾ ⛾ ⛾ ⛾ ⛾ ⛾
Includes juice/Milk/Soup

Total Fat (Grams)

Total Carbohydrate

Steps (Pedometer):_ _ _ _ _ _ _ _ _ _ _ _

Comments & Resolutions:

©

Sunday

	CALORIES		FAT	CARBS or
	Food	Exercise	Grams	Protein
🙂 BREAKFAST/Exercise				
Snack/Exercise				
🙂 LUNCH				
Snack/Exercise				
🙂 DINNER				
Snack/Exercise				

Sun CALORIE TOTALS				
NET CALORIES (Food Minus Exercise)				

WATER/FLUIDS (CUPS) ⊔ ⊔ ⊔ ⊔ ⊔ ⊔ ⊔ ⊔
Includes juice/Milk/Soup

Total Fat (Grams)
Total Carbohydrate

Steps (Pedometer): _ _ _ _ _ _ _ _ _ _ _
Comments & Resolutions:

©

Day	Net Calories	Fat Grams	Carbohydrates
Monday			
Tuesday			
Wednesday			
Thursday			
Friday			
Saturday			
Sunday			
WEEK'S TOTALS			
DAILY AVERAGES Divide totals by 7			

WEIGHT CHANGE

One week ago: _____

Today: _____

Weight Change: _____

WAIST CHANGE

One week ago: _____

Today: _____

Waist Change: _____

⊘ Transfer daily averages for calories and fat to last page.
⊘ Record body measurements on last page (chest, waist, hips, thighs).

COMMENTS :
_____
_____

GOALS / RESOLUTIONS FOR NEXT WEEK:
_____
_____
_____

©

Monday

	CALORIES		FAT	CARBS or
	FOOD	EXERCISE	GRAMS	PROTEIN
☺ **BREAKFAST/Exercise**				
Snack/Exercise				
☺ **LUNCH**				
Snack/Exercise				
☺ **DINNER**				
Snack/Exercise				
Mon **CALORIE TOTALS**				
NET CALORIES (Food Minus Exercise)				

WATER/FLUIDS (CUPS) ▽ ▽ ▽ ▽ ▽ ▽ ▽ ▽
Includes juice/Milk/Soup

Total Fat (Grams)	
Total Carbohydrate	

Steps (Pedometer):_ _ _ _ _ _ _ _ _ _ _ _

Comments & Resolutions:

©

Tuesday

| | CALORIES | | FAT | CARBS |
	FOOD	EXERCISE	GRAMS	or PROTEIN
🙂 BREAKFAST/Exercise				
Snack/Exercise				
🙂 LUNCH				
Snack/Exercise				
🙂 DINNER				
Snack/Exercise				
CALORIE TOTALS				
NET CALORIES (Food Minus Exercise)				

Tue

WATER/FLUIDS (CUPS) ⛢ ⛢ ⛢ ⛢ ⛢ ⛢ ⛢ ⛢
Includes juice/Milk/Soup

| **Total Fat (Grams)** |
| **Total Carbohydrate** |

Steps (Pedometer): _ _ _ _ _ _ _ _ _ _ _

Comments & Resolutions:

©

Wednesday

	CALORIES		FAT	CARBS or
	FOOD	EXERCISE	GRAMS	PROTEIN
☺ BREAKFAST/Exercise				
Snack/Exercise				
☺ LUNCH				
Snack/Exercise				
☺ DINNER				
Snack/Exercise				
Wed CALORIE TOTALS				
NET CALORIES (Food Minus Exercise)				

WATER/FLUIDS (CUPS) ▽ ▽ ▽ ▽ ▽ ▽ ▽ ▽
Includes juice/Milk/Soup

Total Fat (Grams)

Total Carbohydrate

Steps (Pedometer): _ _ _ _ _ _ _ _ _ _

Comments & Resolutions:

PAGE 38 ©

Thursday

	CALORIES		FAT	CARBS or
	Food	Exercise	Grams	Protein
☺ BREAKFAST/Exercise				
Snack/Exercise				
☺ LUNCH				
Snack/Exercise				
☺ DINNER				
Snack/Exercise				
Thu CALORIE TOTALS				
NET CALORIES (Food Minus Exercise)				

WATER/FLUIDS (CUPS) ⛛ ⛛ ⛛ ⛛ ⛛ ⛛ ⛛ ⛛
Includes juice/Milk/Soup

Total Fat (Grams)	
Total Carbohydrate	

Steps (Pedometer):_ _ _ _ _ _ _ _ _ _ _
Comments & Resolutions:

©

Friday

	CALORIES		FAT	CARBS or PROTEIN
	FOOD	EXERCISE	GRAMS	
🙂 BREAKFAST/Exercise				
Snack/Exercise				
🙂 LUNCH				
Snack/Exercise				
🙂 DINNER				
Snack/Exercise				
CALORIE TOTALS				
NET CALORIES (Food Minus Exercise)				

WATER/FLUIDS (CUPS) ▽▽▽▽▽▽▽▽
Includes juice/Milk/Soup

Total Fat (Grams)

Total Carbohydrate

Steps (Pedometer): _ _ _ _ _ _ _ _ _ _ _ _

Comments & Resolutions:

©

Saturday

	CALORIES		FAT	CARBS or PROTEIN
	FOOD	EXERCISE	GRAMS	
☺ BREAKFAST/Exercise				
Snack/Exercise				
☺ LUNCH				
Snack/Exercise				
☺ DINNER				
Snack/Exercise				

Sat	CALORIE TOTALS			
	NET CALORIES (Food Minus Exercise)			

WATER/FLUIDS (CUPS) ▽ ▽ ▽ ▽ ▽ ▽ ▽ ▽
Includes juice/Milk/Soup

Total Fat (Grams)	
Total Carbohydrate	

Steps (Pedometer):_ _ _ _ _ _ _ _ _ _ _

Comments & Resolutions:

©

Sunday

	CALORIES		FAT	CARBS or PROTEIN
	FOOD	EXERCISE	GRAMS	
🙂 **BREAKFAST/Exercise**				
Snack/Exercise				
🙂 **LUNCH**				
Snack/Exercise				
🙂 **DINNER**				
Snack/Exercise				
Sun **CALORIE TOTALS**				
NET CALORIES (Food Minus Exercise)				

WATER/FLUIDS (CUPS) ⛄⛄⛄⛄⛄⛄⛄⛄
Includes juice/Milk/Soup

Total Fat (Grams)
Total Carbohydrate

Steps (Pedometer):_ _ _ _ _ _ _ _ _ _ _

Comments & Resolutions:

©

WEEKLY SUMMARY

week 4

Day	Net Calories	Fat Grams	Carbohydrates
Monday			
Tuesday			
Wednesday			
Thursday			
Friday			
Saturday			
Sunday			
WEEK'S TOTALS			
DAILY AVERAGES Divide totals by 7			

WEIGHT CHANGE

One week ago: _____

Today: _____

Weight Change: _____

WAIST CHANGE

One week ago: _____

Today: _____

Waist Change: _____

⊘ Transfer daily averages for calories and fat to last page.
⊘ Record body measurements on last page (chest, waist, hips, thighs).

COMMENTS : _____

_____

_____

GOALS / RESOLUTIONS FOR NEXT WEEK: _____

_____

_____

_____

Monday

| | CALORIES | | FAT | CARBS or |
	Food	Exercise	Grams	Protein
☺ **BREAKFAST/Exercise**				
Snack/Exercise				
☺ **LUNCH**				
Snack/Exercise				
☺ **DINNER**				
Snack/Exercise				

Mon CALORIE TOTALS				
NET CALORIES (Food Minus Exercise)				

WATER/FLUIDS (CUPS) ▽▽▽▽▽▽▽▽
Includes juice/Milk/Soup

Total Fat (Grams)

Total Carbohydrate

Steps (Pedometer): _ _ _ _ _ _ _ _ _ _

Comments & Resolutions:

©

Tuesday

	CALORIES		FAT	CARBS or
	FOOD	EXERCISE	GRAMS	PROTEIN
☺ BREAKFAST/Exercise				
Snack/Exercise				
☺ LUNCH				
Snack/Exercise				
☺ DINNER				
Snack/Exercise				
CALORIE TOTALS				
NET CALORIES (Food Minus Exercise)				

Tue

WATER/FLUIDS (CUPS) ▽▽▽▽▽▽▽▽
Includes juice/Milk/Soup

Total Fat (Grams)	
Total Carbohydrate	

Steps (Pedometer): _ _ _ _ _ _ _ _ _ _ _ _
Comments & Resolutions:

©

Wednesday

	CALORIES		FAT	CARBS or
	FOOD	EXERCISE	GRAMS	PROTEIN
☺ BREAKFAST/Exercise				
Snack/Exercise				
☺ LUNCH				
Snack/Exercise				
☺ DINNER				
Snack/Exercise				

Wed CALORIE TOTALS		
NET CALORIES (Food Minus Exercise)		

WATER/FLUIDS (CUPS) ▽ ▽ ▽ ▽ ▽ ▽ ▽
Includes juice/Milk/Soup

| **Total Fat (Grams)** |
| **Total Carbohydrate** |

Steps (Pedometer):_ _ _ _ _ _ _ _ _ _ _ _

Comments & Resolutions:

©

Thursday

| | CALORIES | | FAT | CARBS |
	FOOD	EXERCISE	GRAMS	or PROTEIN
☺ BREAKFAST/Exercise				
Snack/Exercise				
☺ LUNCH				
Snack/Exercise				
☺ DINNER				
Snack/Exercise				

| Thu | CALORIE TOTALS | | | |
| | NET CALORIES (Food Minus Exercise) | | | |

WATER/FLUIDS (CUPS) ▽ ▽ ▽ ▽ ▽ ▽ ▽ ▽
Includes juice/Milk/Soup

| Total Fat (Grams) |
| Total Carbohydrate |

Steps (Pedometer):_ _ _ _ _ _ _ _ _ _ _ _

Comments & Resolutions:

©

PAGE 47

Friday

	CALORIES		FAT	CARBS or PROTEIN
	FOOD	EXERCISE	GRAMS	
☺ BREAKFAST/Exercise				
Snack/Exercise				
☺ LUNCH				
Snack/Exercise				
☺ DINNER				
Snack/Exercise				
Fri CALORIE TOTALS				
NET CALORIES (Food Minus Exercise)				

WATER/FLUIDS (CUPS) ▽▽▽▽▽▽▽▽
Includes juice/Milk/Soup

Total Fat (Grams)

Total Carbohydrate

Steps (Pedometer):_ _ _ _ _ _ _ _ _ _

Comments & Resolutions:

©

Saturday

| | CALORIES | | FAT | CARBS or |
	FOOD	EXERCISE	GRAMS	PROTEIN
☺ **BREAKFAST**/Exercise				
Snack/Exercise				
☺ **LUNCH**				
Snack/Exercise				
☺ **DINNER**				
Snack/Exercise				

Sat CALORIE TOTALS				
NET CALORIES (Food Minus Exercise)				

WATER/FLUIDS (CUPS) ⛆ ⛆ ⛆ ⛆ ⛆ ⛆ ⛆ ⛆
Includes juice/Milk/Soup

| **Total Fat (Grams)** | |
| **Total Carbohydrate** | |

Steps (Pedometer): _ _ _ _ _ _ _ _ _ _

Comments & Resolutions:

©

Sunday

	CALORIES		FAT	CARBS or
	Food	Exercise	Grams	Protein
🙂 **BREAKFAST/Exercise**				
Snack/Exercise				
🙂 **LUNCH**				
Snack/Exercise				
🙂 **DINNER**				
Snack/Exercise				

Sun	CALORIE TOTALS			
	NET CALORIES (Food Minus Exercise)			

WATER/FLUIDS (CUPS) ▽ ▽ ▽ ▽ ▽ ▽ ▽ ▽
Includes juice/Milk/Soup

Total Fat (Grams)

Total Carbohydrate

Steps (Pedometer): _ _ _ _ _ _ _ _ _ _ _

Comments & Resolutions:

©

Day	Net Calories	Fat Grams	Carbohydrates
Monday			
Tuesday			
Wednesday			
Thursday			
Friday			
Saturday			
Sunday			
WEEK'S TOTALS			
DAILY AVERAGES Divide totals by 7			

WEIGHT CHANGE

One week ago: _____

Today: _____

Weight Change: _____

WAIST CHANGE

One week ago: _____

Today: _____

Waist Change: _____

⊘ Transfer daily averages for calories and fat to last page.
⊘ Record body measurements on last page (chest, waist, hips, thighs).

COMMENTS :

_____

_____

_____

GOALS / RESOLUTIONS FOR NEXT WEEK:

_____

_____

_____

_____

©

Monday

| | CALORIES | | FAT | CARBS or |
	Food	Exercise	Grams	Protein
🙂 **BREAKFAST/Exercise**				
Snack/Exercise				
🙂 **LUNCH**				
Snack/Exercise				
🙂 **DINNER**				
Snack/Exercise				

	CALORIE TOTALS			
Mon NET CALORIES (Food Minus Exercise)				

WATER/FLUIDS (CUPS) 🥤🥤🥤🥤🥤🥤🥤🥤
Includes juice/Milk/Soup

| **Total Fat (Grams)** | |
| **Total Carbohydrate** | |

Steps (Pedometer):_ _ _ _ _ _ _ _ _ _ _ _

Comments & Resolutions:

PAGE 52

©

Tuesday

	CALORIES		FAT	CARBS or PROTEIN
	FOOD	EXERCISE	GRAMS	
🙂 BREAKFAST/Exercise				
Snack/Exercise				
🙂 LUNCH				
Snack/Exercise				
🙂 DINNER				
Snack/Exercise				
CALORIE TOTALS				
Tue **NET CALORIES** (Food Minus Exercise)				

WATER/FLUIDS (CUPS) ▽▽▽▽▽▽▽▽
Includes juice/Milk/Soup

Total Fat (Grams)

Total Carbohydrate

Steps (Pedometer): _ _ _ _ _ _ _ _ _ _

Comments & Resolutions:

©

Wednesday

	CALORIES		FAT	CARBS or
	FOOD	EXERCISE	GRAMS	PROTEIN
🙂 BREAKFAST/Exercise				
Snack/Exercise				
🙂 LUNCH				
Snack/Exercise				
🙂 DINNER				
Snack/Exercise				
CALORIE TOTALS				
NET CALORIES (Food Minus Exercise)				

WATER/FLUIDS (CUPS) ∇ ∇ ∇ ∇ ∇ ∇ ∇
Includes juice/Milk/Soup

| **Total Fat (Grams)** | |
| **Total Carbohydrate** | |

Steps (Pedometer):_ _ _ _ _ _ _ _ _ _ _

Comments & Resolutions:

PAGE 54

©

Thursday

	CALORIES		FAT	CARBS or PROTEIN
	FOOD	EXERCISE	GRAMS	
😊 BREAKFAST/Exercise				
Snack/Exercise				
😊 LUNCH				
Snack/Exercise				
😊 DINNER				
Snack/Exercise				
CALORIE TOTALS				
Thu NET CALORIES (Food Minus Exercise)				

WATER/FLUIDS (CUPS) ⊔ ⊔ ⊔ ⊔ ⊔ ⊔ ⊔ ⊔
Includes juice/Milk/Soup

Total Fat (Grams)

Total Carbohydrate

Steps (Pedometer):_ _ _ _ _ _ _ _ _ _ _

Comments & Resolutions:

©

Friday

	CALORIES		FAT	CARBS or
	FOOD	EXERCISE	GRAMS	PROTEIN
😊 BREAKFAST/Exercise				
Snack/Exercise				
😊 LUNCH				
Snack/Exercise				
😊 DINNER				
Snack/Exercise				
CALORIE TOTALS				
NET CALORIES (Food Minus Exercise)				

WATER/FLUIDS (CUPS) ▽ ▽ ▽ ▽ ▽ ▽ ▽ ▽
Includes juice/Milk/Soup

Total Fat (Grams)

Total Carbohydrate

Steps (Pedometer):_ _ _ _ _ _ _ _ _ _ _

Comments & Resolutions:

©

Saturday

	CALORIES		FAT	CARBS or
	Food	Exercise	Grams	Protein
☺ **Breakfast**/Exercise				
Snack/Exercise				
☺ **Lunch**				
Snack/Exercise				
☺ **Dinner**				
Snack/Exercise				
Sat CALORIE TOTALS				
NET CALORIES (Food Minus Exercise)				

WATER/FLUIDS (CUPS) ▽▽▽▽▽▽▽▽
Includes juice/Milk/Soup

Total Fat (Grams)

Total Carbohydrate

Steps (Pedometer):_ _ _ _ _ _ _ _ _ _ _

Comments & Resolutions:

©

Sunday

| | CALORIES | | FAT | CARBS or |
	Food	Exercise	Grams	Protein
☺ BREAKFAST/Exercise				
Snack/Exercise				
☺ LUNCH				
Snack/Exercise				
☺ DINNER				
Snack/Exercise				
Sun CALORIE TOTALS				
NET CALORIES (Food Minus Exercise)				

WATER/FLUIDS (CUPS) ▽ ▽ ▽ ▽ ▽ ▽ ▽ ▽
Includes juice/Milk/Soup

Total Fat (Grams)
Total Carbohydrate

Steps (Pedometer): _ _ _ _ _ _ _ _ _ _ _

Comments & Resolutions:

©

WEEKLY SUMMARY

DAY	NET CALORIES	FAT GRAMS	CARBOHYDRATES
Monday			
Tuesday			
Wednesday			
Thursday			
Friday			
Saturday			
Sunday			
WEEK'S TOTALS			
DAILY AVERAGES Divide totals by 7			

WEIGHT CHANGE

One week ago: _____

Today: _____

Weight Change: _____

WAIST CHANGE

One week ago: _____

Today: _____

Waist Change: _____

✓ Transfer daily averages for calories and fat to last page.
✓ Record body measurements on last page (chest, waist, hips, thighs).

COMMENTS : _____
_____
_____

GOALS / RESOLUTIONS FOR NEXT WEEK:
_____
_____
_____

©

Monday

	CALORIES		FAT	CARBS or
	FOOD	EXERCISE	GRAMS	PROTEIN
🙂 BREAKFAST/Exercise				
Snack/Exercise				
🙂 LUNCH				
Snack/Exercise				
🙂 DINNER				
Snack/Exercise				

Mon

CALORIE TOTALS	
NET CALORIES (Food Minus Exercise)	

WATER/FLUIDS (CUPS) ▽ ▽ ▽ ▽ ▽ ▽ ▽ ▽
Includes juice/Milk/Soup

Total Fat (Grams)	
Total Carbohydrate	

Steps (Pedometer): _ _ _ _ _ _ _ _ _ _ _ _

Comments & Resolutions:

©

Tuesday

	CALORIES		FAT	CARBS or
	Food	Exercise	Grams	Protein
☺ BREAKFAST/Exercise				
Snack/Exercise				
☺ LUNCH				
Snack/Exercise				
☺ DINNER				
Snack/Exercise				
CALORIE TOTALS				
Tue NET CALORIES (Food Minus Exercise)				

WATER/FLUIDS (CUPS) ▽ ▽ ▽ ▽ ▽ ▽ ▽ ▽
Includes juice/Milk/Soup

Total Fat (Grams)

Total Carbohydrate

Steps (Pedometer): _ _ _ _ _ _ _ _ _ _ _ _

Comments & Resolutions:

©

Wednesday

| | CALORIES | | FAT | CARBS or |
	Food	Exercise	Grams	Protein
☺ **BREAKFAST**/Exercise				
Snack/Exercise				
☺ **LUNCH**				
Snack/Exercise				
☺ **DINNER**				
Snack/Exercise				

	CALORIE TOTALS		
Wed NET CALORIES (Food Minus Exercise)		

WATER/FLUIDS (CUPS) ▽▽▽▽▽▽▽▽
Includes juice/Milk/Soup

Total Fat (Grams)
Total Carbohydrate

Steps (Pedometer):_ _ _ _ _ _ _ _ _ _ _ _

Comments & Resolutions:

©

Thursday

	CALORIES		FAT	CARBS or
	FOOD	EXERCISE	GRAMS	PROTEIN
☺ BREAKFAST/Exercise				
Snack/Exercise				
☺ LUNCH				
Snack/Exercise				
☺ DINNER				
Snack/Exercise				
Thu CALORIE TOTALS				
NET CALORIES (Food Minus Exercise)				

WATER/FLUIDS (CUPS) ▽ ▽ ▽ ▽ ▽ ▽ ▽ ▽
Includes juice/Milk/Soup

| Total Fat (Grams) |
| Total Carbohydrate |

Steps (Pedometer):_ _ _ _ _ _ _ _ _ _ _

Comments & Resolutions:

©

Friday

	CALORIES		FAT	CARBS or PROTEIN
	FOOD	EXERCISE	GRAMS	
😊 BREAKFAST/Exercise				
Snack/Exercise				
😊 LUNCH				
Snack/Exercise				
😊 DINNER				
Snack/Exercise				
CALORIE TOTALS				
NET CALORIES (Food Minus Exercise)				

WATER/FLUIDS (CUPS) ⛉ ⛉ ⛉ ⛉ ⛉ ⛉ ⛉ ⛉
Includes juice/Milk/Soup

Total Fat (Grams)
Total Carbohydrate

Steps (Pedometer): _ _ _ _ _ _ _ _ _ _ _

Comments & Resolutions:

©

Saturday

	CALORIES		FAT	CARBS or
	FOOD	EXERCISE	GRAMS	PROTEIN
☺ BREAKFAST/Exercise				
Snack/Exercise				
☺ LUNCH				
Snack/Exercise				
☺ DINNER				
Snack/Exercise				

Sat	CALORIE TOTALS			
	NET CALORIES (Food Minus Exercise)			

WATER/FLUIDS (CUPS) ▽ ▽ ▽ ▽ ▽ ▽ ▽ ▽
Includes juice/Milk/Soup

Total Fat (Grams)

Total Carbohydrate

Steps (Pedometer):_ _ _ _ _ _ _ _ _ _ _ _

Comments & Resolutions:

©

Sunday

	CALORIES		FAT	CARBS or
	FOOD	EXERCISE	GRAMS	PROTEIN
😊 BREAKFAST/Exercise				
Snack/Exercise				
😊 LUNCH				
Snack/Exercise				
😊 DINNER				
Snack/Exercise				

	CALORIE TOTALS			
Sun NET CALORIES (Food Minus Exercise)				

WATER/FLUIDS (CUPS) ▽ ▽ ▽ ▽ ▽ ▽ ▽ ▽
Includes juice/Milk/Soup

Total Fat (Grams)

Total Carbohydrate

Steps (Pedometer): _ _ _ _ _ _ _ _ _

Comments & Resolutions:

©

WEEKLY SUMMARY

week 7

DAY	NET CALORIES	FAT GRAMS	CARBOHYDRATES
Monday			
Tuesday			
Wednesday			
Thursday			
Friday			
Saturday			
Sunday			
WEEK'S TOTALS			
DAILY AVERAGES Divide totals by 7			

WEIGHT CHANGE

One week ago: _____

Today: _____

Weight Change: _____

WAIST CHANGE

One week ago: _____

Today: _____

Waist Change: _____

⊘ Transfer daily averages for calories and fat to last page.
⊘ Record body measurements on last page (chest, waist, hips, thighs).

COMMENTS :
_____
_____
_____

GOALS / RESOLUTIONS FOR NEXT WEEK:
_____
_____
_____

Monday

	CALORIES		FAT	CARBS or PROTEIN
	FOOD	EXERCISE	GRAMS	
☺ BREAKFAST/Exercise				
Snack/Exercise				
☺ LUNCH				
Snack/Exercise				
☺ DINNER				
Snack/Exercise				
Mon CALORIE TOTALS				
NET CALORIES (Food Minus Exercise)				

WATER/FLUIDS (CUPS) ▽ ▽ ▽ ▽ ▽ ▽ ▽ ▽
Includes juice/Milk/Soup

Total Fat (Grams)
Total Carbohydrate

Steps (Pedometer): _ _ _ _ _ _ _ _ _ _
Comments & Resolutions:

©

Tuesday

	CALORIES		FAT	CARBS or
	FOOD	EXERCISE	GRAMS	PROTEIN
☺ BREAKFAST/Exercise				
Snack/Exercise				
☺ LUNCH				
Snack/Exercise				
☺ DINNER				
Snack/Exercise				
CALORIE TOTALS				
NET CALORIES (Food Minus Exercise)				

WATER/FLUIDS (CUPS) ☐ ☐ ☐ ☐ ☐ ☐ ☐ ☐
Includes juice/Milk/Soup

Total Fat (Grams)

Total Carbohydrate

Steps (Pedometer):_ _ _ _ _ _ _ _ _ _ _ _

Comments & Resolutions:

©

Wednesday

	CALORIES		FAT	CARBS or
	FOOD	EXERCISE	GRAMS	PROTEIN
😊 **BREAKFAST/Exercise**				
Snack/Exercise				
😊 **LUNCH**				
Snack/Exercise				
😊 **DINNER**				
Snack/Exercise				
Wed **CALORIE TOTALS**				
NET CALORIES (Food Minus Exercise)				

WATER/FLUIDS (CUPS) 🥤🥤🥤🥤🥤🥤🥤🥤
Includes juice/Milk/Soup

Total Fat (Grams)
Total Carbohydrate

Steps (Pedometer):_ _ _ _ _ _ _ _ _ _

Comments & Resolutions:

PAGE 70   ©

Thursday

| | CALORIES | | FAT | CARBS |
	Food	Exercise	Grams	or Protein
☺ **BREAKFAST**/Exercise				
Snack/Exercise				
☺ **LUNCH**				
Snack/Exercise				
☺ **DINNER**				
Snack/Exercise				
Thu **CALORIE TOTALS**				
NET CALORIES (Food Minus Exercise)				

WATER/FLUIDS (CUPS) ▽▽▽▽▽▽▽▽
Includes juice/Milk/Soup

Total Fat (Grams)

Total Carbohydrate

Steps (Pedometer): _ _ _ _ _ _ _ _ _ _ _

Comments & Resolutions:

©

Friday

	CALORIES		FAT	CARBS or PROTEIN
	FOOD	EXERCISE	GRAMS	
☺ BREAKFAST/Exercise				
Snack/Exercise				
☺ LUNCH				
Snack/Exercise				
☺ DINNER				
Snack/Exercise				
Fri CALORIE TOTALS				
NET CALORIES (Food Minus Exercise)				

WATER/FLUIDS (CUPS) ▽ ▽ ▽ ▽ ▽ ▽ ▽ ▽
Includes juice/Milk/Soup

Total Fat (Grams)

Total Carbohydrate

Steps (Pedometer):_ _ _ _ _ _ _ _ _ _ _ _

Comments & Resolutions:

©

Saturday

	CALORIES		FAT	CARBS or
	FOOD	EXERCISE	GRAMS	PROTEIN
🙂 BREAKFAST/Exercise				
Snack/Exercise				
🙂 LUNCH				
Snack/Exercise				
🙂 DINNER				
Snack/Exercise				
Sat CALORIE TOTALS				
NET CALORIES (Food Minus Exercise)				

WATER/FLUIDS (CUPS) ⌷ ⌷ ⌷ ⌷ ⌷ ⌷ ⌷ ⌷
Includes juice/Milk/Soup

Total Fat (Grams)

Total Carbohydrate

Steps (Pedometer):_ _ _ _ _ _ _ _ _ _ _

Comments & Resolutions:

©

Sunday

	CALORIES		FAT	CARBS or PROTEIN
	FOOD	EXERCISE	GRAMS	PROTEIN
🙂 **BREAKFAST/Exercise**				
Snack/Exercise				
🙂 **LUNCH**				
Snack/Exercise				
🙂 **DINNER**				
Snack/Exercise				

Sun	**CALORIE TOTALS**			
	NET CALORIES (Food Minus Exercise)			

WATER/FLUIDS (CUPS) ⛢ ⛢ ⛢ ⛢ ⛢ ⛢ ⛢ ⛢
Includes juice/Milk/Soup

| **Total Fat (Grams)** | |
| **Total Carbohydrate** | |

Steps (Pedometer): _ _ _ _ _ _ _ _ _ _ _

Comments & Resolutions:

©

WEEKLY SUMMARY

Day	Net Calories	Fat Grams	Carbohydrates
Monday			
Tuesday			
Wednesday			
Thursday			
Friday			
Saturday			
Sunday			
WEEK'S TOTALS			
DAILY AVERAGES Divide totals by 7			

WEIGHT CHANGE
One week ago: _____
Today: _____
Weight Change: _____

WAIST CHANGE
One week ago: _____
Today: _____
Waist Change: _____

⊘ Transfer daily averages for calories and fat to last page.
⊘ Record body measurements on last page (chest, waist, hips, thighs).

COMMENTS : _____
_____
_____

GOALS / RESOLUTIONS FOR NEXT WEEK:
_____
_____
_____

©

Monday

| | CALORIES | | FAT | CARBS or |
	FOOD	EXERCISE	GRAMS	PROTEIN
☺ **BREAKFAST/Exercise**				
Snack/Exercise				
☺ **LUNCH**				
Snack/Exercise				
☺ **DINNER**				
Snack/Exercise				

Mon CALORIE TOTALS

NET CALORIES (Food Minus Exercise)

WATER/FLUIDS (CUPS) ▽ ▽ ▽ ▽ ▽ ▽ ▽
Includes juice/Milk/Soup

Total Fat (Grams)
Total Carbohydrate

Steps (Pedometer): _ _ _ _ _ _ _ _ _ _

Comments & Resolutions:

PAGE 76   ©

Tuesday

| | CALORIES | | FAT | CARBS |
	Food	Exercise	Grams	or Protein
☺ **BREAKFAST**/Exercise				
Snack/Exercise				
☺ **LUNCH**				
Snack/Exercise				
☺ **DINNER**				
Snack/Exercise				
CALORIE TOTALS				
True **NET CALORIES** (Food Minus Exercise)				

WATER/FLUIDS (CUPS) ⏣ ⏣ ⏣ ⏣ ⏣ ⏣ ⏣
Includes juice/Milk/Soup

| Total Fat (Grams) | |
| Total Carbohydrate | |

Steps (Pedometer):_ _ _ _ _ _ _ _ _ _ _

Comments & Resolutions:

©

Wednesday

	CALORIES		FAT	CARBS or
	FOOD	EXERCISE	GRAMS	PROTEIN
🙂 **BREAKFAST/Exercise**				
Snack/Exercise				
🙂 **LUNCH**				
Snack/Exercise				
🙂 **DINNER**				
Snack/Exercise				
CALORIE TOTALS				
NET CALORIES (Food Minus Exercise)				

Wed

WATER/FLUIDS (CUPS) ☐ ☐ ☐ ☐ ☐ ☐ ☐ ☐
Includes juice/Milk/Soup

| **Total Fat (Grams)** |
| **Total Carbohydrate** |

Steps (Pedometer): _ _ _ _ _ _ _ _ _ _ _

Comments & Resolutions:

©

Thursday

| | CALORIES | | FAT | CARBS or |
	Food	Exercise	Grams	Protein
☺ BREAKFAST/Exercise				
Snack/Exercise				
☺ LUNCH				
Snack/Exercise				
☺ DINNER				
Snack/Exercise				
Thu CALORIE TOTALS				
NET CALORIES (Food Minus Exercise)				

WATER/FLUIDS (CUPS) ▽ ▽ ▽ ▽ ▽ ▽ ▽ ▽
Includes juice/Milk/Soup

Total Fat (Grams)

Total Carbohydrate

Steps (Pedometer):_ _ _ _ _ _ _ _ _ _ _ _

Comments & Resolutions:

©

Friday

| | CALORIES | | FAT | CARBS or |
	Food	Exercise	Grams	Protein
😊 BREAKFAST/Exercise				
Snack/Exercise				
😊 LUNCH				
Snack/Exercise				
😊 DINNER				
Snack/Exercise				
CALORIE TOTALS				
NET CALORIES (Food Minus Exercise)				

WATER/FLUIDS (CUPS) Includes juice/Milk/Soup 🥤🥤🥤🥤🥤🥤🥤🥤

Total Fat (Grams)

Total Carbohydrate

Steps (Pedometer): _ _ _ _ _ _ _ _ _ _ _

Comments & Resolutions:

©

Saturday

	CALORIES		FAT	CARBS or
	FOOD	EXERCISE	GRAMS	PROTEIN
🙂 BREAKFAST/Exercise				
Snack/Exercise				
🙂 LUNCH				
Snack/Exercise				
🙂 DINNER				
Snack/Exercise				
Sat CALORIE TOTALS				
NET CALORIES (Food Minus Exercise)				

WATER/FLUIDS (CUPS) 〇 〇 〇 〇 〇 〇 〇 〇
Includes juice/Milk/Soup

Total Fat (Grams)	
Total Carbohydrate	

Steps (Pedometer):_ _ _ _ _ _ _ _ _ _ _ _

Comments & Resolutions:

©

Sunday

	CALORIES		FAT	CARBS or
	FOOD	EXERCISE	GRAMS	PROTEIN
☺ **BREAKFAST/Exercise**				
Snack/Exercise				
☺ **LUNCH**				
Snack/Exercise				
☺ **DINNER**				
Snack/Exercise				

CALORIE TOTALS				
Sun **NET CALORIES** (Food Minus Exercise)				

WATER/FLUIDS (CUPS) ▽ ▽ ▽ ▽ ▽ ▽ ▽ ▽
Includes juice/Milk/Soup

Total Fat (Grams)	
Total Carbohydrate	

Steps (Pedometer): _ _ _ _ _ _ _ _ _ _ _

Comments & Resolutions:

©

WEEKLY SUMMARY

week
9

DAY	NET CALORIES	FAT GRAMS	CARBOHYDRATES
Monday			
Tuesday			
Wednesday			
Thursday			
Friday			
Saturday			
Sunday			
WEEK'S TOTALS			
DAILY AVERAGES Divide totals by 7			

WEIGHT CHANGE
One week ago: _____

Today: _____

Weight Change: _____

WAIST CHANGE
One week ago: _____

Today: _____

Waist Change: _____

⊘ Transfer daily averages for calories and fat to last page.
⊘ Record body measurements on last page (chest, waist, hips, thighs).

COMMENTS : _____

_____

_____

GOALS / RESOLUTIONS FOR NEXT WEEK:

_____

_____

_____

©

Monday

| | CALORIES | | FAT | CARBS or PROTEIN |
	FOOD	EXERCISE	GRAMS	
☺ BREAKFAST/Exercise				
Snack/Exercise				
☺ LUNCH				
Snack/Exercise				
☺ DINNER				
Snack/Exercise				
Mon CALORIE TOTALS				
NET CALORIES (Food Minus Exercise)				

WATER/FLUIDS (CUPS) ▽▽▽▽▽▽▽▽
Includes juice/Milk/Soup

| Total Fat (Grams) | |
| Total Carbohydrate | |

Steps (Pedometer): _ _ _ _ _ _ _ _ _ _ _ _

Comments & Resolutions:

©

Tuesday

| | CALORIES | | FAT | CARBS or |
	FOOD	EXERCISE	GRAMS	PROTEIN
🙂 **BREAKFAST**/Exercise				
Snack/Exercise				
🙂 **LUNCH**				
Snack/Exercise				
🙂 **DINNER**				
Snack/Exercise				
	CALORIE TOTALS			
Tue NET CALORIES (Food Minus Exercise)				

WATER/FLUIDS (CUPS) ▽ ▽ ▽ ▽ ▽ ▽ ▽ ▽
Includes juice/Milk/Soup

| **Total Fat (Grams)** | |
| **Total Carbohydrate** | |

Steps (Pedometer):_ _ _ _ _ _ _ _ _ _ _

Comments & Resolutions:

©

Wednesday

	CALORIES		FAT	CARBS or
	FOOD	EXERCISE	GRAMS	PROTEIN
☺ BREAKFAST/Exercise				
Snack/Exercise				
☺ LUNCH				
Snack/Exercise				
☺ DINNER				
Snack/Exercise				
Wed CALORIE TOTALS				
NET CALORIES (Food Minus Exercise)				

WATER/FLUIDS (CUPS) ∇∇∇∇∇∇∇∇
Includes juice/Milk/Soup

Total Fat (Grams)	
Total Carbohydrate	

Steps (Pedometer):_ _ _ _ _ _ _ _ _ _ _

Comments & Resolutions:

©

Thursday

	CALORIES		FAT	CARBS or PROTEIN
	FOOD	EXERCISE	GRAMS	
😊 BREAKFAST/Exercise				
Snack/Exercise				
😊 LUNCH				
Snack/Exercise				
😊 DINNER				
Snack/Exercise				
Thu CALORIE TOTALS				
NET CALORIES (Food Minus Exercise)				

WATER/FLUIDS (CUPS) ▽ ▽ ▽ ▽ ▽ ▽ ▽ ▽
Includes juice/Milk/Soup

| **Total Fat (Grams)** |
| **Total Carbohydrate** |

Steps (Pedometer): _ _ _ _ _ _ _ _ _ _ _ _

Comments & Resolutions:

©

Friday

	CALORIES		FAT	CARBS or PROTEIN
	FOOD	EXERCISE	GRAMS	PROTEIN
😊 BREAKFAST/Exercise				
Snack/Exercise				
😊 LUNCH				
Snack/Exercise				
😊 DINNER				
Snack/Exercise				
Fri CALORIE TOTALS				
NET CALORIES (Food Minus Exercise)				

WATER/FLUIDS (CUPS) ⬜ ⬜ ⬜ ⬜ ⬜ ⬜ ⬜ ⬜
Includes juice/Milk/Soup

Total Fat (Grams)	
Total Carbohydrate	

Steps (Pedometer): _ _ _ _ _ _ _ _ _ _ _ _

Comments & Resolutions:

©

Saturday

	CALORIES		FAT	CARBS or PROTEIN
	FOOD	EXERCISE	GRAMS	
☺ BREAKFAST/Exercise				
Snack/Exercise				
☺ LUNCH				
Snack/Exercise				
☺ DINNER				
Snack/Exercise				
Sat CALORIE TOTALS				
NET CALORIES (Food Minus Exercise)				

WATER/FLUIDS (CUPS) ▽▽▽▽▽▽▽▽
Includes juice/Milk/Soup

Total Fat (Grams)
Total Carbohydrate

Steps (Pedometer): _ _ _ _ _ _ _ _ _ _ _ _
Comments & Resolutions:

©

Sunday

| | CALORIES | | FAT | CARBS or |
	Food	Exercise	Grams	Protein
😊 **BREAKFAST/Exercise**				
Snack/Exercise				
😊 **LUNCH**				
Snack/Exercise				
😊 **DINNER**				
Snack/Exercise				
Sun **CALORIE TOTALS**				
NET CALORIES (Food Minus Exercise)				

WATER/FLUIDS (CUPS) ▽▽▽▽▽▽▽
Includes juice/Milk/Soup

Total Fat (Grams)
Total Carbohydrate

Steps (Pedometer): _ _ _ _ _ _ _ _ _ _

Comments & Resolutions:

PAGE 90   ©

WEEKLY SUMMARY

Day	Net Calories	Fat Grams	Carbohydrates
Monday			
Tuesday			
Wednesday			
Thursday			
Friday			
Saturday			
Sunday			
WEEK'S TOTALS			
DAILY AVERAGES Divide totals by 7			

WEIGHT CHANGE

One week ago: _____

Today: _____

Weight Change: _____

WAIST CHANGE

One week ago: _____

Today: _____

Waist Change: _____

⊘ Transfer daily averages for calories and fat to last page.
⊘ Record body measurements on last page (chest, waist, hips, thighs).

COMMENTS : _____
_____
_____

GOALS / RESOLUTIONS FOR NEXT WEEK: _____
_____
_____

©

MINI CALORIE, FAT & CARB COUNTER

BEVERAGES, COFFEE	CAL	FAT	Cb
Cocoa Mix, 1 oz	100	1	88
Coffee, black, 1 cup	4	0	1
Caffe Latte (nonfat milk), 12 oz	110	0.5	15
Cappuccino (nonfat milk), 12 oz	60	0	9
Tea, black, 1 cup	2	0	0
Iced Tea, sweetened, 8 fl.oz	80	0	20

Tea/Coffee Additions:	CAL	FAT	Cb
Milk: whole, 2 Tbsp, 1fl.oz	20	1	1
Low-fat, 2 Tbsp, 1 fl.oz	16	0	4
Nonfat, 2 Tbsp, 1 fl.oz	5	0	1
Cream: Light, 2 Tbsp, 1fl.oz	60	6	1
½ & ½, 2 Tbsp	40	4	1
Creamers: Liquid, 2 Tbsp	40	2	5
Powdered, 2 tsp	16	1	1.5
Sugar, 1 rounded tsp	24	0	6
Fruit Juice, average, 8 fl.oz	110	0	22
Soft Drinks, average: 8 fl.oz	100	0	25
12 fl. oz	160	0	40
Low Calorie (sugar-free)	1	0	0
Water: Plain/Mineral/Soda	0	0	0

ALCOHOL	CAL	FAT	Cb
Beer, regular, 12 fl.oz	150	0	17
Light Beer, average, 12 fl.oz	110	0	6
Wine, average, 1 glass 4 fl.oz	85	0	2
Sherry, dry, 2 fl.oz	65	0	0.5
Wine Cooler, average, 6 fl.oz	100	0	17
Champagne, 1 glass, 4 fl.oz	85	0	2
Brandy, Vodka, Rum, 1 fl.oz	65	0	0

MILK & MILK DRINKS	CAL	FAT	Cb
Milk: Whole,1 cup 8 fl.oz	150	8	12
Reduced Fat (2% fat),1 cup	120	5	12
Low-fat (1%) 1 cup, 8 fl.oz	100	2.5	12
Fat Free 1 cup, 8 fl.oz	90	0.5	12
Soy Milk, avg., 1 cup, 8 fl.oz	150	5	14

YOGURT: Average All Brands	CAL	FAT	Cb
Plain/Natural, whole, 8 oz	180	7	11
Nonfat, 8 oz	110	0	18
Flavored/Fruited, reg., 8 oz	250	6	38
Low-fat, 8 oz	230	3	32
Nonfat, 8 oz	150	0	32
Nonfat, no sugar, 8 oz	120	0	30

EGGS	CAL	FAT	Cb
1 large, 2 oz	75	5	0
Fried, 1 large, 2 oz	100	8	0
Omelet, 2 eggs, plain	230	19	1

CHEESE	CAL	FAT	Cb
Hard Cheese, average, 1 oz	110	9	0.5
Kraft Light, average,1 oz	60	3	3
Cottage, creamed, 4 oz	120	4	4
Low-fat, 4 oz	80	0.5	4
Cream Chse: Reg, 2 T., 1 oz	100	10	1
Light (Philadelphia) 1 oz	70	5	2
Processed, average, 1 oz	100	8	2
Parmesan, 1 oz	110	7	1
Ricotta, part skim, 4 oz	160	10	4

ICECREAM/ICES: Per ½ Cup	CAL	FAT	Cb
Icecream: Regular (10% fat)	130	7	16
Rich/Premium (16% fat)	170	10	17
Ice Milk, low-fat, ½ cup	100	3	15
Frozen Yogurt, nonfat	110	0	29
Sherbet, 2% fat, ½ cup	120	2	28
Tofu Frozen Desserts, avg.	150	7	19
Sorbet (fruit), average	120	0	30
Popsicle, regular	50	0	12

FATS & OILS, MAYO	CAL	FAT	Cb
Butter: Regular, 1 tsp	35	4	0
1 Tbsp	100	11	0
Whipped, 1 Tbsp	75	8	0
Margarine: Regular, 1 tsp	35	4	0
1 Tbsp	100	11	0
Light, 1 Tbsp	50	6	0
Oils: All edible types, 1 tsp	35	4	0
1 Tbsp	120	14	0
Mayonnaise: Regular, 1Tbsp	100	11	0
Light, 1 Tbsp	50	5	1
Fat-Free (Kraft/Wt.Watch), 1 T.	10	0	3

CREAM: Light Sour,1 Tbsp	20	2	1.5
Half & Half, average, 1 Tbsp	20	2	0.5
Whipping: Heavy, 1 Tbsp	50	5.5	1
Whipped, 1 Tbsp	25	3	0.5

SALAD DRESSINGS: Per 1 Tbsp	CAL	FAT	Cb
French/Italian Dressing: avg.	70	7	2
Light, average, 1 Tbsp	60	5	4
Blue Chse, Thousand Island	50	5	1
Light, average, 1 Tbsp	40	4	0.5
Coleslaw, regular	75	6	5
Ranch, regular	80	8	2

RICE & SPAGHETTI	CAL	FAT	Cb
Rice: Boiled, ½ cup, 3¼ oz	120	0	27
Fried, ½ cup	160	5	21
Spaghetti: Dry, 1 oz	105	0.5	21
Cooked, 1 cup, 5 oz	160	0.5	7

MINI CALORIE, FAT & CARB COUNTER

▶ **MEATS:** *(Cooked, No Added Fat)*

Average all cuts:	CAL	FAT	Cb
Very Lean, 4 oz	160	8	0
Moderate Fat, 4 oz	280	22	0
Fatty, 4 oz	400	35	0
Hamburger Patty, avg., 3 oz	240	17	0
Stew, lean, 1 cup	220	16	1
Lamb Chop, lean, 1 only	160	7	0
Roast Leg, lean, 3 oz	140	6	0
Bacon: Reg, ckd., 3 sl. ¾ oz	110	9	0
Canadian, ckd, 2 sl., 1½ oz	85	8	0
Ham: Roast Leg, lean, 3 oz	150	8	0
Veal: Roast, 2 slices, 3 oz	230	14	0

▶ **SAUSAGES:** *Average all types cooked*

1 small link, ½ oz	50	4	1.5
1 medium link, 1 oz	100	8	2.5
1 large link, 2 oz	150	12	3.5
Frankfurter, avg., 1½ oz	135	12	1

▶ **COLD MEATS**

Bologna, 1 slice, 1 oz	90	8	1
Corned Beef: Canned, 1 oz	65	4.5	1
Fresh, medium fat, 1 oz	105	7.5	0
Ham: Cooked, fresh:			
Lean + fat, 1 oz	90	6	0
Lean only, 1 oz	60	4	0
Canned, average, 1 oz	40	2	0.5
Pastrami, 1 oz	40	2	0.5
Paté, average, 1 oz	60	4	2
Pepperoni, average, 1 oz	140	13	0
Salami: Beef/Beer/Cotto, 1 oz	70	6	0.5
Hard, Genoa, 1 oz	110	10	0.5

▶ **CHICKEN**

Roasted/Microwaved (No Added Fat)

¼ chicken, with skin	230	13	0
no skin	170	6	0
KFC: Original, Thigh	360	25	12
Spicy Crispy Strips, (3)	335	15	23

▶ **FISH**

Low-fat (white flesh):			
Broiled, 1 fillet, 4 oz	130	1	0
Breaded/Batter., fried, 5 oz	320	16	27
Canned: Tuna in Water			
half of 6½ oz can	210	1	0
Tuna in Oil, 6½ oz can	490	42	0
Salmon, ¼ cup, 2 oz	80	4	0
Sardines in Oil, 3¾ oz can, dr.	190	11	0

▶ **FRUIT**

	CAL	FAT	Cb
Apple, 1 medium	90	0	23
Apricot, 1 medium	25	0	6
Avocado, ½ small	90	9	3.5
Banana, 1 medium	80	0	18
Berries, average, ½ cup	40	0	10
Cherries, sweet, 10 only	40	0	10
Grapefruit, 1 medium	40	0	10
Grapes, 4 oz bunch	70	0	15
Melon-Cantaloup, ¼ medium	45	0	11
Nectarine, 1 medium	50	0	12
Orange, 1 medium	80	0	20
Peach, 1 large, 6 oz	55	0	13
Pear, 1 small, 4 oz	60	0	15
Pineapple, 1 slice, 3 oz	40	0	10
Plum, 1 medium, 3 oz	45	0	11
Strawberries, 1 cup, 5½ oz	45	0	11
Watermelon, ½ sl., 1" thick	50	0	12
Dried Fruit: average, 1 oz	80	0	20

▶ **VEGETABLES**

Asparagus, 4 spears, 2 oz	15	0	3
Beans, Snap, ½ cup, 2 oz	20	0	4
Beets, 1 whole, 4 oz	35	0	4
Broccoli, ckd, ½ cup, 3 oz	25	0	5
Cabbage, ckd, ½ cup, 2½ oz	15	0	2
Carrot, ckd, ½ cup, 2½ oz	35	0	8
Cauliflower, ckd, ½ cup, 3 oz	15	0	3
Celery, 6" piece, 1 oz	4	0	1
Corn: Cob, 3½" ear	60	1	14
Kernels, ½ cup, 2¾ oz	65	1	14
Cucumber, 6 slices, 2 oz	5	0	1
Lettuce, 2 leaves, 1 oz	2	0	0.5
Onion, 1 medium, 4 oz	40	0	9
Peas, green, raw, ½ c., 3 oz	70	0	12
Peppers, sweet, 1 only, 3 oz	20	0	5
Potato: Small, 3 oz	65	0	15
Fries, 3" fried, 10 only	160	8	9
Oven-heated, 10 only	105	4	12
Hash Browns, ½ c., 2½ oz	165	10	10
Pumpkin, ckd, ½ cup, 4 oz	25	0	6
Tomato, 1 medium, 5 oz	35	0	8

▶ **NUTS & SEEDS**

Nuts, average, 20 nuts, 1 oz	170	15	5
Sunflower Kernels, dried, 1 T.	50	4	3.5

MINI CALORIE, FAT & CARB COUNTER

▶ BREAKFAST CEREALS	CAL	FAT	Cb
All Bran, 1/2 cup, 1 oz	80	1	23
Branflakes, 3/4 cup, 1 oz	90	1	18
Cornflakes, 1 cup, 1 oz	110	0	24
Granola Natural, 1/4 cup	110	4.5	16
Oatmeal, ckd, 3/4 cup, 6 oz	110	2	22
Puffed Rice, 1 cup, 1/2 cup	60	0.5	12
Raisin Bran, 1/2 cup	85	0	20

▶ BREAD			
Average: 1 thin slice, 1 oz	70	1	13
1 thick slice, 1 1/2 oz	105	1.5	20
Toast: Same Cals & Fat as bread used			
1 thin slice + 2 tsp fat	140	9	13
Bread Rolls, Dinner	85	2	15
Hamburger Bun, 1 1/2 oz	120	2	23
Bagel, plain, 3" diam.	160	1.5	30
Croissant, plain, lrg, 2 1/2 oz	300	18	35
Pita, 1 small, 2 oz	150	2	30
Pumpernickel, 1 oz	75	1	15

▶ SANDWICHES			
BLT	600	46	46
Chicken Salad w. Mayo	580	30	49
Club Sandwich	830	38	31
Corned Beef on Rye	560	28	44
Cream Cheese and Jelly	350	14	46
Egg Salad w. Mayo	570	29	49
Ham Salad	320	17	30
Hot Dog	310	13	39
Peanut Butter and Jelly	370	25	28
Roast Beef + Mustard	460	12	45
Tuna Salad w. Mayo	610	30	49

▶ SPREADS, PRESERVES			
Honey, 2 tsp	50	0	12
Jam, Preserves, avg, 2 tsp	40	0	10
Jelly Marmalade, avg, 2 tsp	40	0	10
Low Calorie, average, 2 tsp	4	0	1
Ham Spread, 1 tsp	35	0.5	0
Peanut Butter, 1 T., 1/2 oz	105	8.5	3.5

▶ CRACKERS: Per Cracker			
Cheese, 1" square, each	5	0.1	1
Sandwich type, p/nut butter	200	10	23
Graham, Plain, 2	30	1	5
Matzo, 6" square	115	2	25
Saltines, 1 square	12	0.5	2
Wheat, thin	9	0.2	1
Whole-wheat	15	0.2	3

▶ CAKES & PASTRIES	CAL	FAT	Cb
Apple Pie, 4 oz	290	13	46
Carrot Cake w. Frosting 4 oz	400	21	46
Cheesecake, plain, 3 oz	260	18	24
Choc. Cake w. Icing, 2 oz	235	12	26
Croissant, plain, 2 1/2 oz	300	18	35
Donut: Glazed, 2 oz	250	12	34
Iced/Chocolate, average	260	14	29
Fruit Cake, 1 1/2 oz	165	7	26
Muffin, blueberry, medium	240	9	36
Pancake: Plain, average, 4"	80	3	11
Lower Calorie, 4"	45	1	8
Pecan Pie, 4 oz	470	24	52
Plain Cake, no frosting, 3 oz	310	12	42
Sponge Cake, plain, 2 1/2 oz	190	3	36

▶ COOKIES: Sweet, plain, 1	55	2	7
Chocolate Chip, each	80	4	10
Oreo, regular, each	55	2.5	7
Peanut Butter, each	70	4	7
Shortbread, each	75	5	7
Mrs Fields, average, each	280	14	40

▶ DESSERTS			
Custard, average, 1/2 cup	120	5.5	11
Gelatin Dessert, 1/2 cup	80	0	18
Low Calorie, 1/2 cup	8	0	2
Rice Pudding, can., 3 1/2 oz	160	7.5	22
Waffle, 2 1/2 oz	245	13	26

▶ CANDY			
Chocolate: Solid, 1 oz	150	10	15
w. Fruit/Nuts, 1 oz	150	10	15
Choc Bar/Kit Kat, 1 1/2 oz	215	12	27
Carob-coated Bar, av, 1 1/2 oz	225	15	23
Fudge, Choc. or Nuts 1 oz	120	4	21
Gum, Chewing, avg., 1 only	8	0	2
Bubble Gum, 1 only	25	0	6
Hard Candy, 1 piece	18	0	5
M&M's, plain, 1.7 oz pkt	240	10	34
Mars Bar, 1.8 oz	240	13	31

▶ SNACK FOODS			
Beef Jerky, average, 1 oz	70	1	0
Cheese Curls, 1 1/4 cup, 1 oz	160	9	19
Corn Chips, av, 1 oz pkt	160	10	15
Granola Bar, average, 1 oz	130	2.5	26
Nuts, average, 1 oz	170	15	5
Potato Chips, 1 oz packet	150	10	15
Popcorn, no oil, plain, 1 cup	20	0	4
Pretzels, average, 1 oz	110	2	22
Tortilla Chips, 1 oz packet	150	8	22

MINI CALORIE, FAT & CARB COUNTER

▶ ARBY'S	CAL	FAT	Cb
Arby-Q	360	14	40
Chicken Caesar Salad (no dr.)	230	8	8
Grilled Chicken Deluxe	450	22	37
Hot Ham 'N' Swiss S'wich	340	13	35
Junior Roast Beef	290	12	34
Roast Chicken Club	520	28	39
Regular Roast Beef	450	21	48
Turkey Sub	630	37	51

▶ BURGER KING	CAL	FAT	Cb
Burgers: Hamburger	310	14	30
Cheeseburger	360	17	31
Whopper, with Cheese	805	50	53
Veggie Burger	340	10	47
Chicken Caesar Salad (no dr.)	160	6	5
Chicken Baguettes, avg.	350	4	47
Croissan'wich w. Egg/Chse	320	19	24
French Fries, small	230	11	29
Fish Fillet Sandwich	520	30	44
Shake, small, average	620	32	72

▶ DAIRY QUEEN	CAL	FAT	Cb
Chicken Breast Fillet	430	20	37
Grilled Chicken s/which	310	10	30
Hamburger	290	12	29
Double Cheeseburger	540	31	30
Hot Dogs: Regular	240	14	19
Cone: Small, average	230	7	38

▶ DENNY'S	CAL	FAT	Cb
Choc Layer Cake, 3 oz	275	12	42
Grilled Chicken Dinner	130	4	0
Gr. Chicken S'wich (no fries)	480	14	53
Garden Deluxe Salad w/Chkn Breast (no dressing or bread)	230	11	10
Rst Turkey & Stuffing/Gry	365	3	38
Slim Slam, no topping	440	6	56
Orig. Grand Slam B'fast	1030	60	101
Side Garden Salad (no dress)	115	4	16

▶ HARDEE'S	CAL	FAT	Cb
Bacon Egg & Cheese Biscuit	520	30	45
Burgers: Famous Star	570	35	41
Hamburger	270	10	29
Hot Ham'n'Cheese	300	12	34

▶ KFC	CAL	FAT	Cb
Chicken Breast:Orig. Recipe	370	19	11
Extra Crispy	470	28	19
Hot & Spicy	505	29	23
Kentucky Nuggets, 6 pces	285	18	15
Hot Wings, 6 pces	470	33	18
Potato Wedges, 4.8 oz	375	15	53

▶ JACK IN THE BOX	CAL	FAT	Cb
Breakfast Jack	310	14	33
Hamburger	310	14	30
Chicken Faijita Pita	330	11	35

▶ McDONALD'S	CAL	FAT	Cb
Egg McMuffin	300	12	29
Burgers: Big N' Tasty	530	32	37
Big Mac	580	33	47
Cheeseburger	330	14	36
Hamburger	280	10	35
Chicken McGrill	400	17	37
Filet-o-Fish	470	26	45
McChicken	430	23	41
McGriddles (Bac/Egg/Chse)	450	23	43
McVeggie Burger	350	8	47
Quarter Pounder	430	21	37
Chkn Caesar Salad (no dress)	210	7	11
Spanish Omelete Bagel	710	40	59

▶ PIZZA HUT: *Medium Pizza- Per Slice*	CAL	FAT	Cb
Thin n' Crispy: Cheese	210	9	22
Pepperoni	200	9	21
Veggie Lover's	190	7	24
Pan Pizza: Cheese	285	14	28
Pepperoni	280	14	28
Veggie Lover's	270	12	30
Personal Pan: Ham	595	23	70

▶ SUBWAY: *'7 Under 6' Sandwiches (6")* (Does not include cheese, mayo or oil)	CAL	FAT	Cb
Ham; Roast Beef	290	5	46
Roasted Chicken Breast	320	5	45
Subway Club®	325	6	46
Turkey Breast	280	4	46
Veggie Delite®	225	3	44

▶ TACO BELL: Taco, reg.	170	10	13
Soft Taco: Beef	210	10	20
Chicken	190	6	19
Taco Salad w/Salsa(no Shell)	410	21	33
Gordita Baja™ Beef	360	19	31
Burrito Supreme, Beef	440	18	50

▶ WENDY'S	CAL	FAT	Cb
Chicken BLT Salad(no dress)	315	16	10
Chicken Breast Fillet S/wich	434	16	46
Grilled Chicken s/which	305	7	36

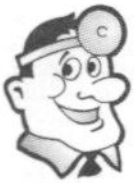

10 Week Progress CHART

WEEK	WEIGHT	AVERAGE CALORIES	AVERAGE FAT/GRAMS	MEASUREMENTS			
				Chest	Waist	Hips	Thigh
START							
1							
2							
3							
4							
5							
6							
7							
8							
9							
10							

~ PROGRESS SUMMARY ~

DATE: ____________ **TOTAL WEIGHT LOSS:** ____________

TOTAL INCHES/CMS LOST: Chest ____________ **Waist** ________

Hips ____________ **Thigh** ________

BODY FAT(%): Start ____________ **Finish** ____________

GOAL WEIGHT NEXT 10 WEEKS: ________ ***(Start Another Diary)***

BLOOD PRESSURE: Date ____________ **Reading** ________

Date ____________ **Reading** ________

BLOOD CHOLESTEROL: Date ____________ **Level** ________

Date ____________ **Level** ________